Merry Christmas '99

MEDITATION

MADE EASY

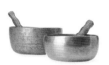

*Wishing you
the best for the
coming year.*

Ruth

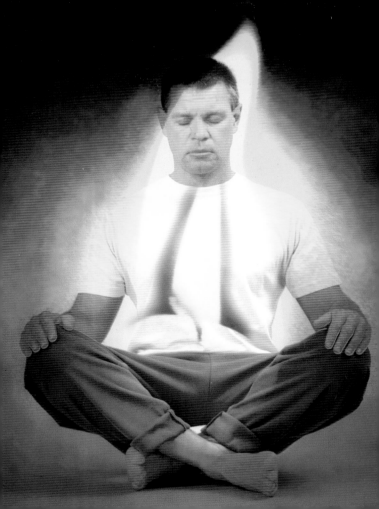

MEDITATION

MADE EASY

Gerry Maguire Thompson

GODSFIELD PRESS

10 9 8 7 6 5 4 3 2 1

Published in 1999 by
Sterling Publishing Company, Inc.
387 Park Avenue South,
New York, N.Y. 10016

Distributed in Canada by
Sterling Publishing
c/o Canadian Manda Group,
One Atlantic Avenue, Suite 105
Toronto, Ontario, Canada M6K 3E7
Distributed in Australia by
Capricorn Link (Australia) Pty Ltd
P O. Box 6651, Baulkham Hills,
Business Centre, NSW 2153, Australia

Printed and bound in Hong Kong

Sterling ISBN 0-8069-9909-8

Library of Congress Catloguing-in-Publication Data
Maguire Thompson, Gerry, 1950—
    Meditation made easy : an introduction to the basics
of the ancient art of meditation/Gerry Maguire Thompson.
        p.   cm.
    Includes index.
    ISBN 0 -8069-9909-8
BL627.C73   1999
    158. 1'2--dc21
                                        99-20346
                                        CIP

ACKNOWLEDGMENTS
*The publishers wish to thank the following
for the use of pictures:*
Bridgeman Art Library: 56
Sally & Richard Greenhill:
6, 7, 15, 48, 50
Images: 36, 42, 42–43, 66,
67, 70, 71, 72, 73
Impact: 79
Science Photo Library: 64
Werner Forman: 26, 27, 34, 35, 44

Illustrations:
Lorraine Harrison, Ivan Hissey

Photography:
Ian Parsons

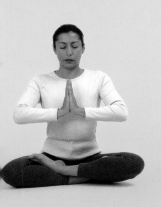

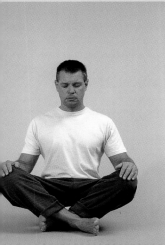

Contents

Introduction

The hectic pace and relentless pressures of modern life are leading more and more people to turn to the art of meditation. This ancient practice has given untold millions

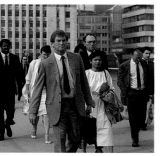

the ability to detach themselves from their problems and gain a clearer perspective and all-round improvement in their quality of life.

Meditation Made Easy is a clear and simple introduction

Above: **Modern-day life can bring stresses, and many people seek relief in meditation.**

to this subject. It is ideal for total beginners, as well as those who may have dabbled in the past and would now like to apply a more systematic approach. Realistic about how people run their lives today, thi straightforward and accessible book takes the reader step by step through all the natural stages of learning to meditate. It demystifies the more esoteric aspects of the subject, and places

Above: The Sanskrit word for *aoum*, the supreme Hindu mantra used for meditation.

emphasis on practicality, enabling the reader to make definite progress by spending as little as ten minutes a day on basic meditation.

The book goes on to give guidance on developing the practice farther, and offers a comprehensive introduction to a wide variety of more specific meditation methods.

Left: Ten minutes a day of basic meditation can offer you all sorts of benefits, from increasing concentration to improving long-term health.

How to Use This Book

This book is divided into four sections. The first section gives some useful background information and explains why meditation can be such a powerful and valuable addition to your lifestyle.

The second section gets you started in a very practical way. It gives advice for those starting from scratch, provides details on how to set up arrangements

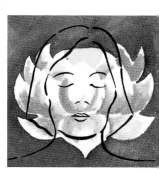

Above: This book helps you to develop your own methods of meditation, which may, for example, include visualization.

for meditation, and outlines a very simple form of meditation practice, step by step. Most newcomers will get the best results by staying with one such simple practice for at least a few weeks, before experimenting with other forms.

The third section offers a variety of more specific types of meditation. This section is not necessarily intended to be taken sequentially, but can be dipped into according to personal needs and preferences.

The last section of this book shows you how to continue enjoying meditation and farther integrate it into your daily life in order to gain the maximum possible benefit.

INTRODUCTORY
TEXT SUMMARIZING
THE SUBJECT

PRACTICAL
PHOTOGRAPHY

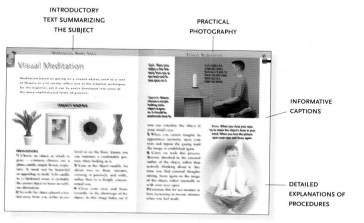

INFORMATIVE
CAPTIONS

DETAILED
EXPLANATIONS OF
PROCEDURES

Why Meditate?

The regular practice of meditation has an extraordinarily wide range of benefits because it exerts a powerful influence on the workings of the mind. The mind in untutored operation has an alarming potential for busyness. The mind in single-pointed focus, by contrast, is calm, efficient, and orderly. The person who can use the mind in the latter way is able to deal with one thing at a time, rather than being overwhelmed by a plethora of demands. This ability enables us to function more efficiently.

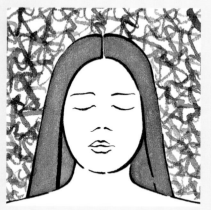

Above: A calm, focused mind is the aim of meditation. It improves our ability to achieve results.

THE BENEFITS OF MEDITATION

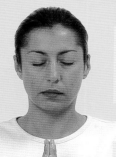

✓reducing the effects of emotional problems, such as panic attacks

✓producing beneficial chemicals known as endorphins and enhancing overall mood

✓reducing brain activity to the relaxed alpha state, bringing increased relaxation and calmness

✓improving efficiency, by enabling you to focus on one task at a time

✓enabling detachment from stressful sources of worry

✓helping with respiratory problems and improving breathing

✓bringing both immediate short-term results as you practice and more profound long-term benefits as you continue

✓normalizing blood pressure and other heart and circulation functions

The History of Meditation

Meditation has been around for a very long time. It has been present in almost all forms of religions and spiritual customs, from highly evolved Tibetan Tantric Buddhism to the simple contemplative practices of the early Christians.

Ironically, as the world we live in today is becoming increasingly hectic, we are all the more in need of something that will help restore this placid quality.

Twenty or thirty years ago, the Eastern act of meditation was little known in the West. Since then, however, its increase in popularity has been extraordinary, with teachers of meditation and centers of teaching becoming established in most cities and even small towns.

Above: **This sacred temple banner originating from Tibet has been used as a meditational aid for centuries.**

Left: **Meditation is traditionally associated with the Orient and has recently spread to the West.**

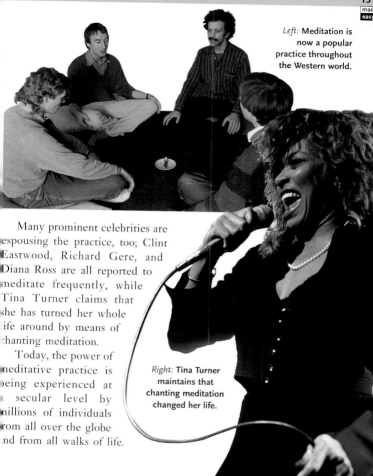

Left: **Meditation is now a popular practice throughout the Western world.**

Many prominent celebrities are espousing the practice, too; Clint Eastwood, Richard Gere, and Diana Ross are all reported to meditate frequently, while Tina Turner claims that she has turned her whole life around by means of chanting meditation.

Today, the power of meditative practice is being experienced at a secular level by millions of individuals from all over the globe and from all walks of life.

Right: **Tina Turner maintains that chanting meditation changed her life.**

The Essence of Meditation

Meditative practices vary a great deal, yet they share a number of common aspects. Whatever form it takes, meditation involves consciously persuading the mind to work in a controlled manner, usually by bringing it to bear on a chosen subject favored by the practitioner.

However down-to-earth or even sophisticated a particular practice is, meditation is a way of training the mind to behave differently from its usual involuntary manner.

THE MIND CAUSING STRESS

The workings of the mind itself, when left unchecked, will actually manufacture problems for us. How much time, for instance, do you

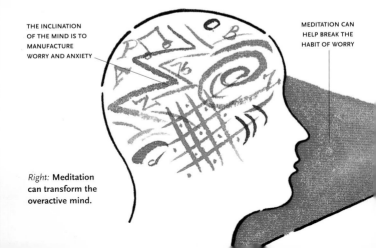

THE INCLINATION OF THE MIND IS TO MANUFACTURE WORRY AND ANXIETY

MEDITATION CAN HELP BREAK THE HABIT OF WORRY

Right: **Meditation can transform the overactive mind.**

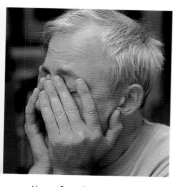

Above: **If we allow our minds to function unchecked, we can create unnecessary worry.**

spend worrying about something that has happened in the past, even though you know there is nothing you can do about it? How often do you panic about an issue that may come up in the future, even when there is little you can do about it now? How often have you despaired in anticipation of something that after all never actually happened?

The fundamental essence of meditation is to focus the mind, let go of our worries, and be fully in the present moment.

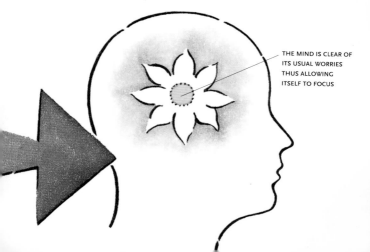

THE MIND IS CLEAR OF ITS USUAL WORRIES THUS ALLOWING ITSELF TO FOCUS

Starting to Meditate

Even the most basic form of meditation can bring great benefits. In fact, the simplest forms are probably the most powerful, and the most venerated.

To start with, short periods of meditation are by far the best. A regular daily practice of just five or ten minutes will be of far more

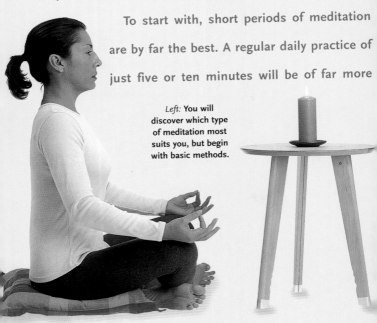

Left: You will discover which type of meditation most suits you, but begin with basic methods.

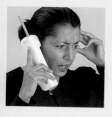

Above: **Modern communications are just one of the many stresses with which we have to contend.**

value than a longer period squeezed in only occasionally. Putting aside a regular time each day is also helpful. If you do this, your body and mind will soon become accustomed to the practice and you will begin to feel the benefits, which will naturally enable you to practice for longer if you so wish.

Some people feel that they are too busy to meditate at all. There is an interesting paradox here. If you get into the habit of setting aside even a little time each day for a simple meditation routine, the result is that the day seems longer and you will manage to get more done.

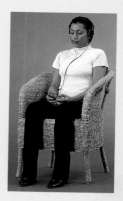

Right: **Always try to meditate, whatever your surroundings. You'll be surprised how easily it fits into your routine.**

Preparing to Meditate

It is important to take time over your preparations before sitting down to meditate, in order to be comfortable, reduce distractions, and increase the benefits obtained. Here are some key aspects to consider.

• Choose a time during the day when you will be undisturbed. Disconnect the phone.

• It is better to meditate when you feel fresh rather than tired.

• Wait for at least two hours after eating a main meal.

• Pick a reasonably quiet location, which can be indoors or outside, depending on your preference.

• Make sure you will be warm enough, but not overly hot.

• Decide how long you are going to meditate, and put a clock or watch within view.

• Sit in a position that enables you to have your spine straight and comfortable for the length of time chosen. This may be in an upright chair – a soft armchair is unsuitable – or on the floor.

• If you are seated on the floor, it is usually necessary to raise the buttocks with sufficient cushions to enable you to sit up straight without effort.

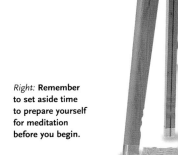

HAVE A CLOCK
WITHIN VIEW

Right: **Remember to set aside time to prepare yourself for meditation before you begin.**

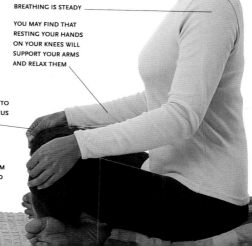

ALTERNATIVE POSTURES

The classic meditation pose is to sit cross-legged on the floor but many people find this uncomfortable, especially for long periods of time. There are plenty of other postures to choose from. You may prefer to sit in a simple, upright chair (keeping your back straight and your feet flat on the floor, as shown here). If you are having difficulty finding a comfortable position, wedge cushions beneath you.

SHOULDERS SHOULD BE RELAXED BACK SO THAT THE CHEST OPENS UP AND YOUR BREATHING IS STEADY

YOU MAY FIND THAT RESTING YOUR HANDS ON YOUR KNEES WILL SUPPORT YOUR ARMS AND RELAX THEM

TRY TO KEEP YOUR HANDS RELAXED UNLESS YOU WANT TO USE THEM AS A FOCUS FOR MEDITATION

MATTING WILL PREVENT YOU FROM FEELING THE COLD

Simple Meditation

On the following pages you will find a simple, classic meditative technique, together with a number of variations on this method. The description includes many generic guidelines and principles that apply to all forms of meditation.

Remember that "simple" does not mean inferior, since the single most valuable principle is to remove the mind from its habitual complex and hyperactive way of working.

PROCEDURE FOR BREATH-CENTERED, BASIC MEDITATION

1 Allow yourself to relax. In your mind, check around your body to see if you are holding muscular tension anywhere, and consciously let go of it.

2 Let go of any concerns that may be in your mind, about what you have just been doing or what you will be doing later.

3 Bring your mental attention to the breath. Take a few long, slow, deep breaths, then let the breath

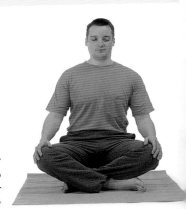

Above: **When you are sitting comfortably, concentrate your mind on your breathing.**

settle into its own pattern. Breathe slowly and easily, in and out through the nose. Try to let the breath flow naturally, rather than making it happen.

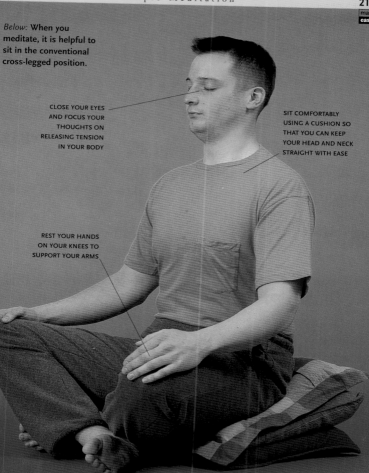

Below: When you meditate, it is helpful to sit in the conventional cross-legged position.

CLOSE YOUR EYES AND FOCUS YOUR THOUGHTS ON RELEASING TENSION IN YOUR BODY

SIT COMFORTABLY USING A CUSHION SO THAT YOU CAN KEEP YOUR HEAD AND NECK STRAIGHT WITH EASE

REST YOUR HANDS ON YOUR KNEES TO SUPPORT YOUR ARMS

4 Bring the attention of your mind to the physical point where the breath is entering and leaving your body, which you will feel in the facial area behind the nose. Focus consciously on this point, and simply observe the cycle of varying sensation as the breath enters and leaves.

5 Inevitably, you will in due course notice that your mind has drifted from your breathing and is

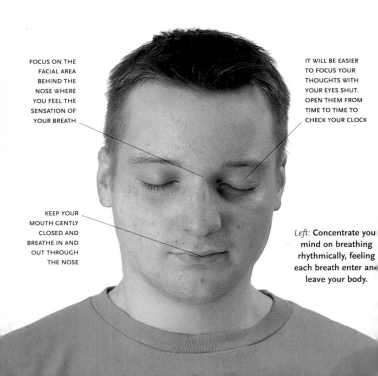

FOCUS ON THE FACIAL AREA BEHIND THE NOSE WHERE YOU FEEL THE SENSATION OF YOUR BREATH

IT WILL BE EASIER TO FOCUS YOUR THOUGHTS WITH YOUR EYES SHUT. OPEN THEM FROM TIME TO TIME TO CHECK YOUR CLOCK

KEEP YOUR MOUTH GENTLY CLOSED AND BREATHE IN AND OUT THROUGH THE NOSE

Left: **Concentrate you mind on breathing rhythmically, feeling each breath enter an leave your body.**

busily wondering what you can have for dinner, and so on. Don't worry about this – simply notice it, and gently bring your attention back to your breathing.

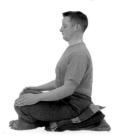

Above: **When it is time to finish your meditation, bring your mind back to your body and how it is feeling.**

6 From time to time you may need to check your clock and return to the meditation. When the time is up, bring your attention back to the whole body and how it is feeling now. Slowly move from your sitting position, and stretch gently.

7 After your period of meditation, try to retain this relaxed state of mind as you go about your next activity. It is as simple as that.

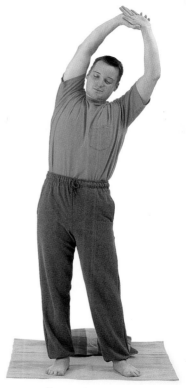

Above: **At the end of the session, slowly rise from your sitting position and do some gentle stretches.**

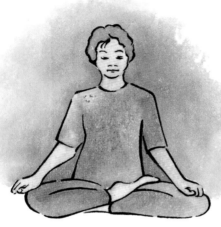

Left: **The yoga lotus position is believed to enhance concentration. Concerns about what is happening in your life will disappear as you focus your thoughts.**

VARIATIONS

The same basic method can also be used, substituting alternative objects for the focus of the mind.

• The attention can be focused on another part of the breathing system, such as the throat or the tip of the nose.

• Alternatively, you could focus your attention on another part of the body altogether, such as the middle of the abdomen or the center of the chest.

The basic goal of this practice is to focus the mind away from the external pressures of everyday life, at the same time letting go of any tension that is being held in any part of your body.

When you practice meditation regularly, you will inevitably become more able to free yourself from the habitual patterns of the mind, and will gradually move toward a more calm and happy overall life state.

AREAS ON WHICH TO FOCUS ATTENTION

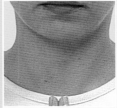

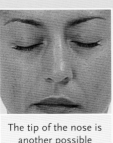

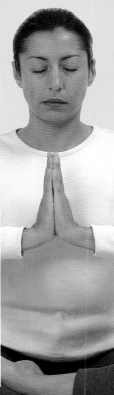

You may choose to focus on another part of the breathing system such as the throat.

The tip of the nose is another possible point of focus when concentrating on in- and out-breaths.

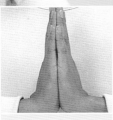

Alternatively, you could focus on a particular part of your body such as the abdomen.

Cupping the hands together in prayer against the chest may help you focus on this area.

Specialized Meditations

This section provides an introduction to a number of more specialized meditation practices. There is a great variety of meditation techniques that have evolved in different cultures and for different purposes. Some are straightforward and easy to get the hang of, while others take a certain degree of practice. Some make use of the sense of sound; others focus on vision, smell, or even taste.

The immediate goals of these different methods also vary widely – from being calming to being energizing; from developing awareness to changing negative habits of thought; from creating

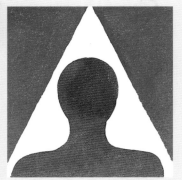

Above: **Meditation depends very much on the individual mind and personal preferences.**

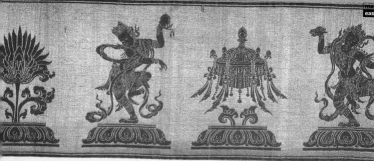

compassion to becoming more focussed; from physical healing to developing one's highest human potential.

Above: This Sino-Tibetan altar cloth pictures auspicious emblems and *puja devis* who offer gifts to the Buddhas of meditation.

Here is a brief introduction to the most popular examples of these specialized techniques. You can follow the directions that were given in the previous section on simple meditation and use any of the standard sitting positions, unless instructed otherwise. Any of the practices that follow may be started with a few minutes of relaxed sitting in your preferred form of breath-centered basic meditation (see p.20).

Sensory Awareness Meditation

This is one of the purest forms of meditation, a classic technique known in the East as *"Vipassana."* The aim is to enter a state of mind whereby you are aware of but detached from all the thoughts that you are experiencing.

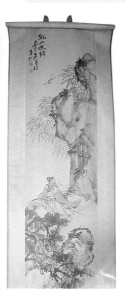

The essence of this practice is to focus upon and allow into your consciousness whatever comes up – emotions, thoughts, plans, worries, fantasies, and so on – and observe them in a detached way, rather than being bound up with them by examining pros and cons and action – as is the custom with everyday mental processes.

Left: This Chinese painting, dating back to 1900, portrays a meditating poet beneath a cliff.

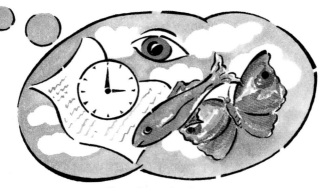

Above: Abstract thoughts may enter your head, some peaceful, others more pressured.

PROCEDURE

1 Sit in a position that you find comfortable with your back straight but relaxed. Keep your eyes half-open and focus on a spot on the floor a few feet in front of you.

2 Simply notice your experiences as each moment passes. When you become aware that you are caught up in a particular train of thought, set of feelings, or mental scenario, simply acknowledge that this has taken place and let it go.

3 Wait and see what comes up next, and treat it in the same way.

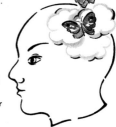

Right: When a particular image appears in your mind, let it travel quietly through and make way for the next image.

4 With practice, you will cultivate openness of the mind and the ability to let go of the habit of always judging or evaluating thoughts. If you catch yourself having this kind of preferential reaction – "this is good, that is bad, I wish the other wasn't true" – simply notice it, then let it go.

5 If you find that certain feelings or thought patterns are becoming particularly distracting, revert to

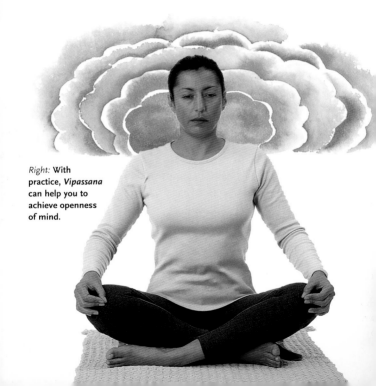

Right: **With practice, *Vipassana* can help you to achieve openness of mind.**

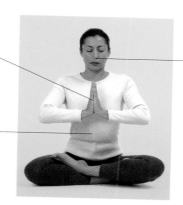

TRADITIONALLY, THE PRAYER POSE SIGNIFIES A JOINING OF THE INDIVIDUAL AND THE DIVINE SOUL

AT THE END OF THE SESSION, BRING YOUR THOUGHTS BACK TO YOUR BREATHING

YOUR BACK SHOULD BE STRAIGHT BUT THERE SHOULD BE NO TENSION HELD HERE OR ANYWHERE ELSE IN YOUR BODY

Left: As with any type of meditation, choose a position you find comfortable and conducive to calm.

breath-centered basic meditation (see p.20) until you feel calm and centered again.

6 Finish the session by bringing your awareness back to the breath and the body, and remain seated for a few more minutes before getting up and doing some gentle stretches and continuing with the rest of your day.

It may take some commitment and practice to master this method. It is highly effective for those who tend to feel swept this way and that – thrown off-center by life's ups and downs.

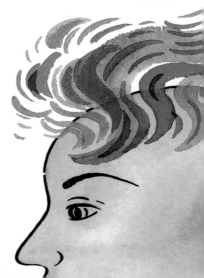

Loving Kindness Meditation

This is one of the great classic practices of Buddhism. However, it may be used to advantage by anyone, whether spiritually oriented or not. Use it to develop a more positive way of looking at life or to bring peace to a certain situation.

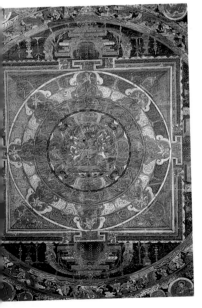

This form of meditation is an exercise in generating focussed compassion, traditionally called "Metta." It benefits not only the meditator but also people around him or her. Many people also use it to help create forces for global peace and positive thinking.

PROCEDURE

1 Sit in a comfortable position with your eyes closed, and bring your attention to the breath. Allow the body to relax, and if you feel any tension in the body, imagine it disappearing as you breathe out. When you are ready to begin the exercise, take a full in-breath.

Left: This sacred Tibetan temple banner depicts a mandala, the Buddhists' perfected universe.

Right: **First concentrate on dispelling negative thoughts, then focus on drawing positive energy into your chest. Finally, as you breathe out, imagine feelings of love flowing from your being.**

2 As you breathe out, imagine releasing and expelling negative emotions such as anger, wishing harm to another person, criticizing yourself, or feeling a failure. As you breathe in again, imagine the positive energies of the universe – such as kindness, generosity, forgiveness, and love – flowing into your body. Continue this with each outward breath for a few minutes, until you feel more positively oriented.

3 Now focus your attention inwardly on the center of your upper chest – this is the center of compassionate emotion. Breathe into this point, and as you do so experience those positive energies flowing into this area. As you breathe out, direct these energies into feelings of loving kindness that flow outward from this center of your being.

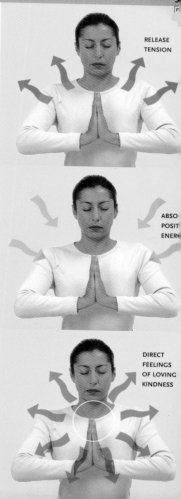

RELEASE
TENSION

ABSO
POSIT
ENER

DIRECT
FEELINGS
OF LOVING
KINDNESS

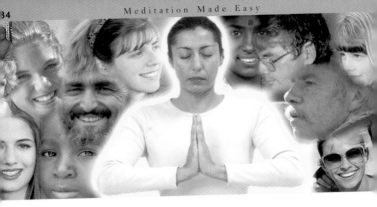

4 Continue to send out this loving kindness in a number of stages. First of all, wish well to yourself for a few minutes. Then direct this feeling to someone else, about whom you feel very positive or loving; then to someone you feel quite neutral about, or don't know very well; then to someone whom you positively resent or feel negative about. Stay with each of these for a minute or two. Try to visualize these feelings as an actual flow of real energy.

5 Finally, extend this flow of loving kindness to a wider circle of friends, family, and contacts; then to people of your town or

Above and opposite: **End your session by directing loving kindness to a wider group of people starting with your friends (left), and ending with the entire world (right).**

city; then to your country; and finally to the whole world.

6 Finish by bringing your focus back to yourself. Open your eyes, and ground yourself by looking around the room at your surroundings for a few moments.

You may or may not directly experience the feeling of "Metta," or loving kindness at first. But if you practice the stages and are open, you will gradually find that it becomes stronger.

eas

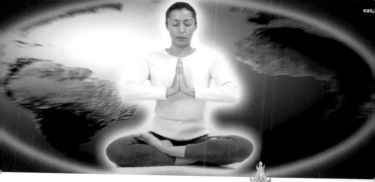

ESHO FUNI

According to the Buddhist principle of "Esho Funi," your own inner sources manifest your experiences from the outer environment. That is why this meditation is one of the most powerful methods of improving relationships, attracting positive reactions from others, having more favorable life experiences, and generally becoming a happier person.

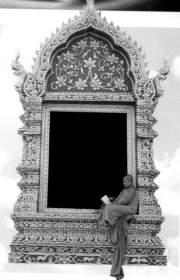

Right: **Buddhists have been exploring the power of meditation for centuries. This Thai monastery was built c. 1296.**

Meditation on Sound

There are two main forms of meditation based on sound. The first involves listening to a sound of your choice, and the second is based on creating the sound yourself. Here are some of the classic examples of each form.

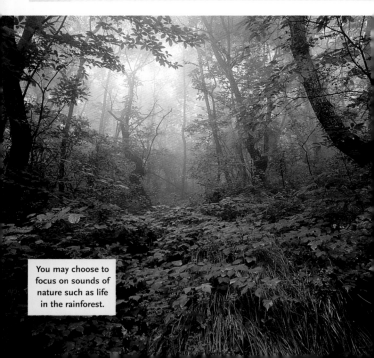

You may choose to focus on sounds of nature such as life in the rainforest.

LISTENING MEDITATION

In this type of practice, the single-pointedness of attention is brought to bear on the sense of hearing, to the exclusion of all the other faculties. For instance, you could choose to listen to

- a music tape or CD
- a recording of natural sounds, such as the ocean or rainforest
- whatever sounds happen to be going on in your surroundings. This may be the breeze in the trees or the sound of a gently flowing stream if you have found a place to meditate outside.

PROCEDURE

1 Sit in a comfortable position, with your eyes closed.

2 Tune your attention to your chosen sound source and listen passively, not analytically. Take in each sound, then let it go, without dwelling on its associations.

3 When other thoughts enter your mind, bring your attention back to whatever sound you are hearing at that particular moment.

INSTRUMENTS OF SOUND

A variation of this form is to use sound sources that you control or create yourself – traditionally these are instruments that are valued for their vibrational or spiritual effect. Examples include oriental gongs, bells, Tibetan cymbals, and singing bowls. The sound source or instrument is sounded intermittently; your attention is placed on the sound, which is then dwelt on in the mind after the sound has died away. When your attention has wandered or the sound cannot be recalled, it is made again.

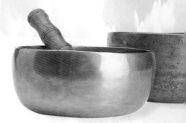

Above: Tibetan singing bowls have been used for centuries as an aid to sound meditation.

VOCAL MEDITATION

Uttering certain sounds has long been considered a powerful way of meditating and creating positive physical and spiritual results, because of the subtle vibrational effect that voiced sound has on the inner energies of the body and the consciousness. The sounds (words or phrases) are called mantras and are repeated continuously. Here is one of the simplest practices, used in many traditions since time immemorial and based on the archetypal sound "Aoum."

PROCEDURE

1 Sit in a comfortable position, taking care that your spine is straight but relaxed. Breathe deeply into the abdomen several times, then let the breath settle into its natural rhythm until you feel calm and centered.

2 Take another breath into the abdomen. Over the whole out-breath, utter the sound sequence A-O-U-M. Repeat this in- and out-breath sequence with the sound several times.

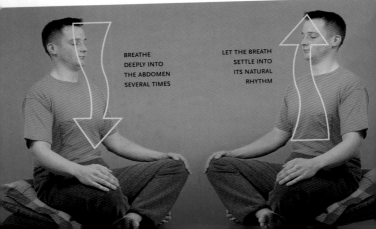

BREATHE DEEPLY INTO THE ABDOMEN SEVERAL TIMES

LET THE BREATH SETTLE INTO ITS NATURAL RHYTHM

THE MOST SACRED MANTRA

This symbol represents the Sanskrit word for "Aoum," a sacred syllable intoned as part of Hindu devotion and contemplation. This meditational technique is widely used by people who also practice yoga. However, anyone wishing to practice mantra meditation may choose any word or sound upon which to focus; your choice may depend on your own personal spiritual beliefs or simply something that you find effective and contemplative.

Below and opposite:
After taking a deep breath, release your breath and utter "A-O-U-M" on the out-breath.

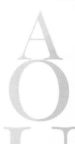

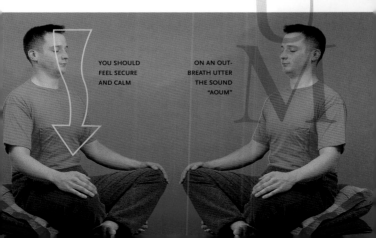

YOU SHOULD
FEEL SECURE
AND CALM

ON AN OUT-
BREATH UTTER
THE SOUND
"AOUM"

3 When you have mastered sounding the syllables, begin to focus on each of the individual components of the sequence, feeling the vibrations they create in your body. On the "A" sound, your attention is on the lower abdomen, and you may notice the vibrational effect in this area. By the time you have reached the "M" sound, the vibrations will be felt in the throat and head.

4 Repeat this sound sequence continuously. After about ten such

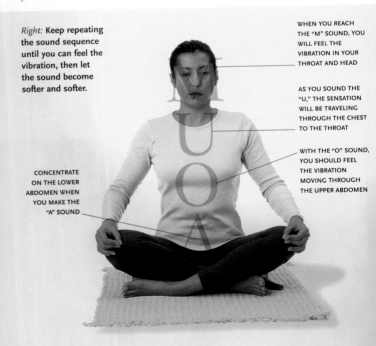

Right: Keep repeating the sound sequence until you can feel the vibration, then let the sound become softer and softer.

WHEN YOU REACH THE "M" SOUND, YOU WILL FEEL THE VIBRATION IN YOUR THROAT AND HEAD

AS YOU SOUND THE "U," THE SENSATION WILL BE TRAVELING THROUGH THE CHEST TO THE THROAT

WITH THE "O" SOUND, YOU SHOULD FEEL THE VIBRATION MOVING THROUGH THE UPPER ABDOMEN

CONCENTRATE ON THE LOWER ABDOMEN WHEN YOU MAKE THE "A" SOUND

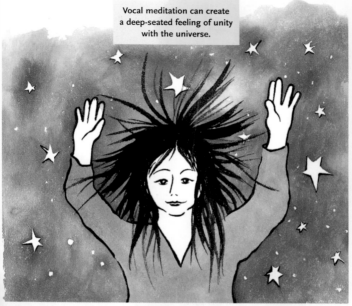

Vocal meditation can create a deep-seated feeling of unity with the universe.

repeats, or when you are feeling the effects more clearly, allow the sound to become gradually softer, until it is not being voiced at all, but only internally imagined.

5 To end the session, bring your attention to your breathing again. Continue sitting for a few minutes, and observe any sensations or effects that are noticeable in your state of being.

This form of meditation can have a powerful effect on raising your personal energies and creating a profound feeling of oneness with the cosmos.

CHANTING MEDITATION

This practice is an even more powerful means of energizing and transforming consciousness than vocal meditation. The precise effects, goals, and purpose of each meditation vary depending on the chosen chanted phrase.

The procedure is similar to that used for vocal meditation, except that the phrase is repeated continuously, drawing breath as necessary, without interrupting the rhythm. The mind is focused either on the syllables themselves or on their content, with the intention of realizing this thought in your own life.

During this form of meditation, try to make each utterance of the phrase conscious and individual, rather than becoming mesmerized into a hypnotic pattern.

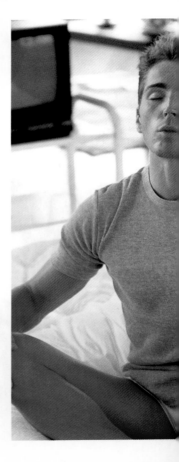

Right: **Assume a comfortable position for meditation and begin chanting the phrase of your choice, concentrating on the words or their meaning.**

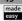

Here are some of the most highly revered chants, together with a brief indication of their meaning:

"Nam-myo-ho-ren-ge-kyo" evokes the latent qualities of the Buddha within each human individual.

"Aoum Mani Padme Hum" means "Hail to the jewel in the lotus."

"Allah Hu" is the Sufi invocation of God.

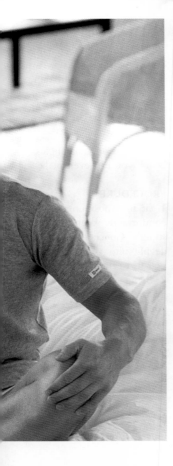

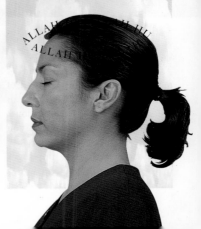

MANTRA MEDITATION

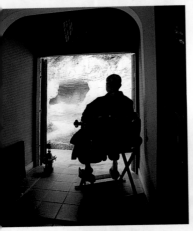

Above: **A Japanese Abbot sits in quiet contemplation of the temple's Zen-style gardens.**

This is a time-honored form of meditation, in which the sound of a particular word is dwelt upon in the mind, but not spoken out loud.

The choice of word that you will use to meditate upon is not necessarily considered important in itself. It can be obtained in a number of ways. It may be

• given to you personally by a teacher or guru, as is usual in Transcendental Meditation.
• a common archetypal word with a meaning that has particular significance for you, such as "peace" or "shalom."
• a random or meaningless word, which you can even make up.

PROCEDURE

1 Sit in a position that you find comfortable, keeping your back straight. Concentrate on breathing deeply into your abdomen, until you feel centered and relaxed.

2 Bring your attention to the mantra, and repeat it inwardly to yourself, in a rhythm with your breath. This can be done either once or twice on each in-breath and each out-breath.

3 When you have settled into the meditation, you may be able to omit the rhythmic repetition and focus instead continuously on the word itself, as a purely surface phenomenon, rather than going

Right: As you breathe in,
repeat your chosen mantra to
yourself, either once or twice.

PEACE

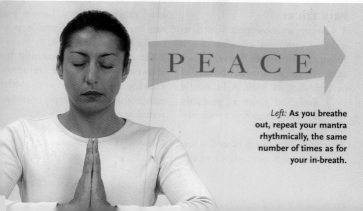

into its meaning in your mind. If
you notice your mind wandering,
bring your thoughts back to the
inner sound of the mantra again.

When you have discovered a
mantra that suits you and with
which you are comfortable, it is
best to use it exclusively, rather
than switching around from one to
another. You may then find it is
useful to repeat your mantra to
yourself a couple of times at
stressful moments in your life, to
restore your inner calm.

PEACE

Left: As you breathe
out, repeat your mantra
rhythmically, the same
number of times as for
your in-breath.

Visual Meditation

Meditation based on gazing on a chosen object, such as a vase of flowers or a lit candle, offers one of the simplest techniques for the beginner, yet it can be easily developed into some of the more sophisticated forms of practice.

OBJECT GAZING

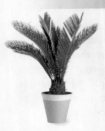 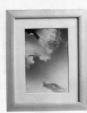 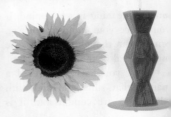

PROCEDURE

1 Choose an object at which to gaze – common choices are a plant, candle, simple flower, or picture. It need not be beautiful or appealing in itself. A lit candle in a darkened room is probably the easiest object to focus on without distraction.

2 Sit with the object placed a few feet away from you, either at eye level or on the floor. Ensure you can maintain a comfortable posture when looking at it.

3 Gaze at the object steadily for about two to three minutes, viewing it passively and softly rather than in a sharply concentrated way.

4 Close your eyes and focus inwardly on the afterimage of the object. As this image fades, see

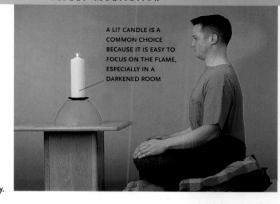

right: Place your object a few feet away from you at eye level and fix your gaze on it.

A LIT CANDLE IS A COMMON CHOICE BECAUSE IT IS EASY TO FOCUS ON THE FLAME, ESPECIALLY IN A DARKENED ROOM

Opposite: Always choose a simple-looking static object to gaze at. It should be positioned close by.

you can visualize the object in your mind's eye.

When you cannot imagine its appearance anymore, open your eyes and repeat the gazing until the image is established again.

Carry on with this process. Become absorbed in the external reality of the object, rather than actively thinking about it. Any time you find external thoughts arising, focus again on the image of the object, either internally or with your eyes open.

Continue this for ten minutes at first, increasing to twenty minutes when you feel ready.

Below: When you close your eyes, try to retain the object's form in your mind. When you lose the picture, open your eyes and focus again.

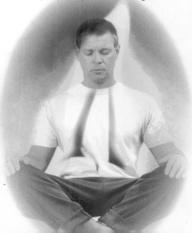

INNER GAZING

As you practice object gazing, you will find that you become more able to grasp an image of the object while you are gazing, and can hold the image in your mind's eye for longer with your eyes closed. Once you have mastered object gazing, you can move on to a meditation where no external object is used, but a significant image is created internally.

Internal imaging is a highly developed practice in such ancient esoteric practices as Tibetan Tantric meditation. Spiritually symbolic images that can be used might include
- the lotus flower
- a mandala (pictorial symbol of the universe)
- the yin–yang symbol
- the image of a deity.

TANTRIC MEDITATION

This is a specialized branch of meditation that involves elaborate techniques. Tantric initiates can take many years of practice to master such methods in their quest for enlightenment.

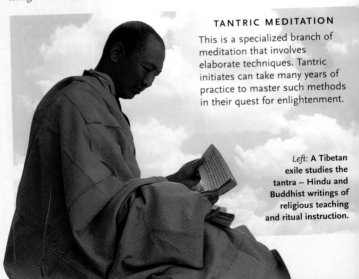

Left: **A Tibetan exile studies the tantra – Hindu and Buddhist writings of religious teaching and ritual instruction.**

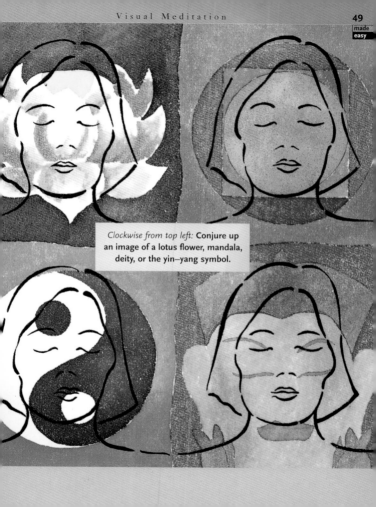

Clockwise from top left: **Conjure up an image of a lotus flower, mandala, deity, or the yin–yang symbol.**

Healing Meditation

Healing meditation works by bringing the power of
visualization to bear internally on the body. It can be used
in a number of different ways — for instance, focusing on a
specific, ailing part of the body, or working more generally
on improving your own overall health and well-being.

SPECIFIC HEALING

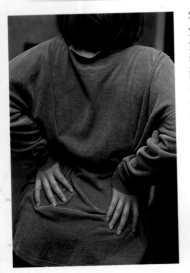

Specific healing is the focus of
your attention on whatever part of
your body system is affected by
ill-health. It might be a painful
joint or bone, a sore area of skin,
an aching muscle, or an internal
organ that is causing trouble such
as ill-functioning kidneys.

The main thing to remember is
to have something specific to focus
on in your mind's eye.

Left: Many people suffer from
back problems, so the back is
a common object of focus for
specific healing. Try to identify
a particular area of discomfort
such as a muscle or a specific
area of the spine.

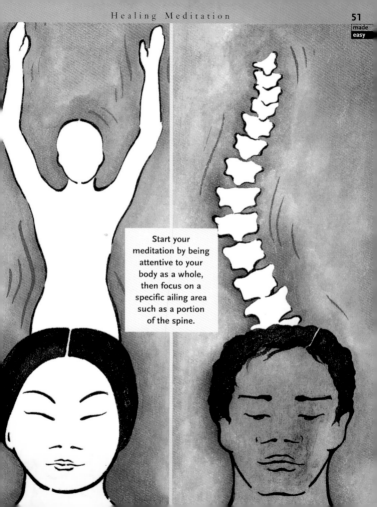

Start your meditation by being attentive to your body as a whole, then focus on a specific ailing area such as a portion of the spine.

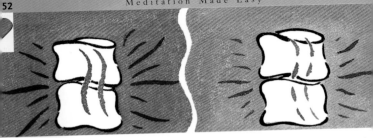

PROCEDURE

1 Sit in a comfortable position with your back straight and your eyes closed. Focus your attention on your breath, until it is regular and you feel centered. Bring your attention to the body as a whole.

2 Now turn your attention to the site of the health problem. See this part of your body in your mind, and notice how it seems to you – you may think of it as physically damaged, darkened or polluted, swollen, or otherwise impaired. Don't worry if you are unsure what the body part looks like in real life – it is your own conceptualization that is important, rather than anatomical accuracy.

3 Picture in your mind's eye the physical or practical processes that would act to remedy the situation – to fix broken bones, realign joints, cool inflammation, clear away infection, and so on. Let any spontaneous images arise naturally in your mind, no matter how simplistic they seem. Cultivate a feeling of loving attention to the task at hand. Continue until you

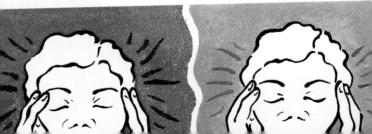

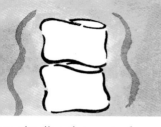

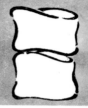

an visualize that part of your
ody system fully healed and in
ristine condition.

Finish by bringing your focus
ack to the whole body. Spend a
ew minutes evaluating how you
eel overall, before opening your
yes, then look around the room
o ground yourself.

bove and below: **When you are focussed
n the ailing part of your body – such as
n area of spine (above) or the position of
migraine (below) – direct feelings of love
o the area while imagining the necessary
ealing processes.**

WHATEVER YOU VISUALIZE IS OKAY

When you visualize the part of
your body you want to heal, you
may imagine it quite differently
from its actual real-life form. It
may appear as a cartoon-style
shape, or it may vary from real
life in its texture or
color. However you
visualize it is fine;
don't get caught
up with trying to
create the image in
anatomical accuracy.

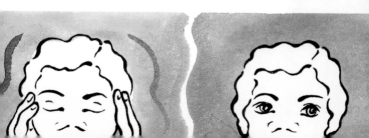

OVERALL HEALING

PROCEDURE

1 Assume a comfortable meditation position, focus on the rhythm of your breathing, and relax.

2 Create in your mind a picture of yourself in perfect health. Explore all the different aspects of this; visualize how you look when you possess abundant energy, a positive mood, a relaxed and supple body, and so on. Go into as much detail as possible.

3 Finish by bringing the attention back to the rhythm of your breath for a few minutes, and see how you now feel in yourself, before opening your eyes and coming back to your surroundings.

VARIATION

An additional element you can include during this practice is to imagine brilliant white light from a surrounding source pervading

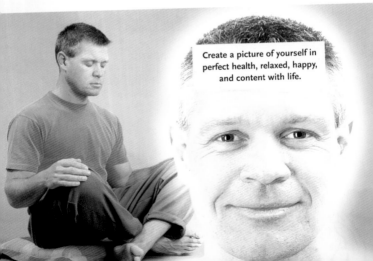

Create a picture of yourself in perfect health, relaxed, happy, and content with life.

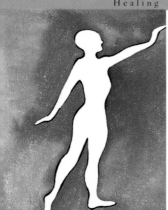

Left: **Imagine a brilliant white light that pervades your whole body, cleansing and healing it.**

your whole body, making its way into its every nook and cranny. Imagine this light flushing out toxicity and leaving your whole body system clear and pure. Then finish the meditation as before.

If you are experiencing clinical depression or mental illness, it may not be appropriate to practice meditation; consult your health practitioner in this case.

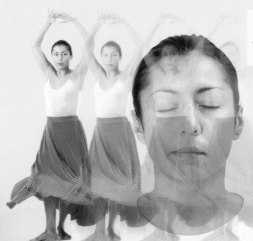

Imagine how your body looks and feels with abundant energy and supple joints.

Chakra Meditation

Chakra meditation focuses on the subtle internal energy
centers of the body — known as chakras — which have been
used for contemplation and spiritual development in both
East and West for thousands of years.

The seven classic chakras lie in a
line through the center of the
trunk of the body, just in front of
the spine. They are usually treated
in sequence from the lowest
upward. If you do not possess
much sense of these centers at
first, begin by visualizing them in
the positions described. With
practice, you will become more
aware of the concentration of
internal energies at these points.

PROCEDURE

1 Sit in a comfortable position,
taking care that the spine is

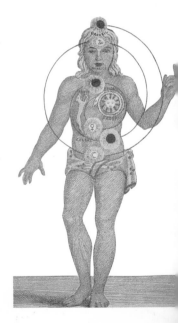

Right: This ancient illustration
from the *Theosophica Practica*
shows the seven chakras and
their position along the trunk
of the physical body.

straight but relaxed. Bring your attention to your breath in the lower abdominal area.

2 Focus your attention on the first chakra, at the base of the spine. Imagine your in-breaths flowing into this point, and your out-breaths flowing out from it. Sense that the chakra is being energized by the external energies brought in by your breath.

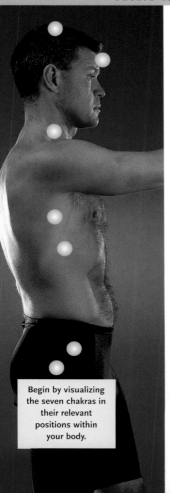

Begin by visualizing the seven chakras in their relevant positions within your body.

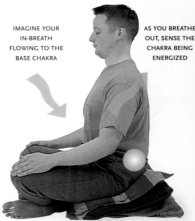

IMAGINE YOUR IN-BREATH FLOWING TO THE BASE CHAKRA

AS YOU BREATHE OUT, SENSE THE CHAKRA BEING ENERGIZED

Above: **Focus on each chakra in turn and imagine your breath flowing to and from it.**

3 After a few minutes, bring your attention to the second chakra, just above the genitals, and follow the same procedure.

4 Continue in this way through the remaining chakras, till you reach the one positioned at the top of your head, the crown. You will probably find that the sense of energy comes less quickly at some of the chakras than at others, because they are blocked or stagnant. If this is the case, give them a little extra time and attention.

5 When you have completed the crown, take your attention briefly to each chakra in turn, from bottom to top, with the image that

you are unblocking the natural energy flow through the whole series, and balancing the energies between them. Then be aware that the base chakra connects you to the earth and the crown chakra to the heavens, and sense the integration of your physical and spiritual energies with the whole of the universe.

This meditation is a powerful way of activating and balancing your personal energies, thereby improving your overall health and feeling of well-being.

Right: **Focus on each chakra individually until you reach the crown, imagining your breaths flowing to and from the particular energy center.**

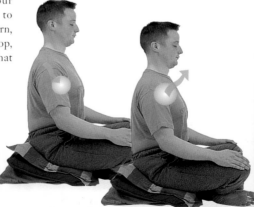

easy

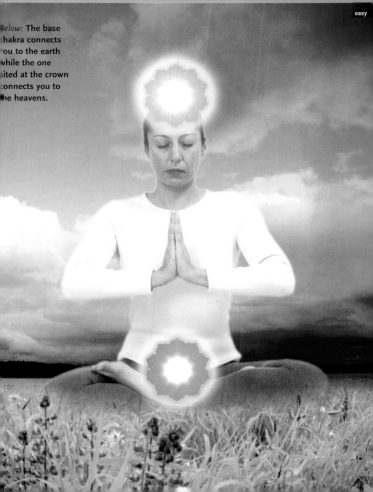

Below: The base chakra connects you to the earth while the one sited at the crown connects you to the heavens.

THE CHAKRAS AND THEIR QUALITIES

Chakras can be seen as complex meeting points of energy, each of which interacts with the others and with the rest of the body. When the chakras are working together coherently, balance is maintained throughout the body. Each chakra is associated with a particular area of the body and with a specific quality (see right). These qualities can be singled out for meditation practice.

CHAKRA TROUBLESHOOTING

chakra	troubles	positive qualities
1	• primitive fears • worry about survival	• *security* • *stability*
2	• sexual weakness • lack of vitality	• *sexual confidence* • *creativity*
3	• lack of confidence • low self-esteem	• *personal power* • *self-worth*
4	• undeservingness • emotional restriction	• *ability to love* • *sense of freedom*
5	• poor communication • loneliness	• *self-expression* • *living in harmony*
6	• lack of imagination • lack of wisdom	• *reliable intuition* • *discernment*
7	• material attachment • mundane existence	• *higher consciousness* • *spiritual purpose*

7: CROWN
Top of head
Higher consciousness

6: BROW
Between eyebrows
Intuition

5: THROAT
Mid-line of throat
Expression

4: HEART
Heart level, central
Love

3: SOLAR PLEXUS
Below breastbone
Power

2: SACRAL
Genitals
Sexuality

1: BASE
Base of spine
Survival

SINGLE CHAKRA MEDITATION

Meditation on any specific chakra can enhance your physical well-being and your potential in the body areas and life functions that the chakra is associated with. You may wish to use this type of meditation for any of the chakras that you habitually find blocked, or for developing qualities that you feel are weak.

CHAKRA COLOR MEDITATION

Chakra meditation can be enhanced by adding color to your visualization. The colors associated with each of the seven chakras are shown on page 65. Here is an example of how to use them.

PROCEDURE

1 Start with the first two steps of chakra meditation (see p.56).
2 Begin to imagine the color red in your mind's eye. Allow the vision of this color to pervade your awareness of the base chakra. Feel the distinctive vibrational quality of the color red, as you continue energizing and breathing into this energy center.
3 When this process is well established, leave the visualization

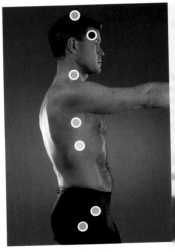

Above: **Each of the seven chakras (see p.61) is associated with a different color.**

nd bring your attention to the
whole body. Finish off by sitting
till for a few minutes, making a
mental note of any sensations and
ffects of the meditation. Open
our eyes, and slowly bring your
ocus back to your surroundings.

This enhanced form of chakra
meditation can be a powerful and
nstantaneous tool for use
when you feel the presence
f particular deficiencies or
weaknesses as you go through life.
For instance, if you find yourself
suddenly feeling threatened or
insecure, the chakra meditation
described above, using the color
red and focusing on the base
chakra (associated with survival),
will be helpful. To improve your
ability to communicate effectively,
use the color blue and focus
on the throat chakra
(related to expression).

ight: **By focusing on
single chakra and
s color you will
ring added power
 your meditation.**

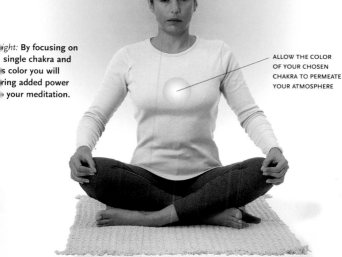

ALLOW THE COLOR
OF YOUR CHOSEN
CHAKRA TO PERMEATE
YOUR ATMOSPHERE

THE CHAKRAS AND THEIR COLORS

The seven chakras are linked to, and stimulated by, the seven color waves of the spectrum, which may be seen when light is passed through a prism or refracted as a rainbow. Meditating on one of these colors, in association with its specific chakra, can help to restore balance to the body and create a state of harmony.

Above: **When light is passed through a prism, it produces a rainbow of seven colors.**

COLOR IMBALANCES

chakra	problem	color
1	lack of will-power, courage, basic fear or worry, low vitality	*red*
2	poor appetite, stagnated energy, inhibition	*orange*
3	low spirits, pessimism, nervous exhaustion	*yellow*
4	headaches, stress, jittery nerves, lack of generosity	*green*
5	insomnia, shock, feverishness, overexcitement	*blue*
6	pain, anger, mental strain, hysteria	*indigo*
7	highly-strung nature, nervous disposition, neurotic tendency	*violet*

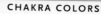

CHAKRA COLORS

Chakra	Color
Base	Red
Sacral	Orange
Solar plexus	Yellow
Heart	Green
Throat	Blue
Brow	Indigo
Crown	Violet

Taking it Farther

The previous section introduced a variety of ways of conducting a meditation session. Now let us look at how the meditative approach can be applied to life in broader terms. This includes a number of possibilities: • using the meditation techniques informally in the course of day-to-day life • applying the principles and approaches of meditation to other everyday activities • enhancing the benefits obtainable from meditation by use of closely associated methods of improving health and well-being.

There are many situations when you can use shortened or adapted versions of the meditation practices already learned. You might wish to practice a shortened method because you find yourself feeling stressed, emotionally disturbed, or thrown off-center at a particular point in your day or because

ou find that an opportunity for meditation arises, when noth-
ng else is happening.

Common situations when an adapted meditation session
an be incorporated include the following • while traveling •
uring a break at work • while standing in line or sitting in a
aiting room • while in a traffic jam.

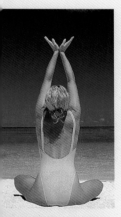

Above: **Regular meditation
and breathing techniques are
an integral part of yoga.**

These informal meditations can
last as long as you wish. In moments
of stress at work, for instance, you
might benefit from a mini-meditation
– bringing your attention to the
breath for as little as twenty or thirty
seconds can often break a cycle of
stress, energizing you with a renewed
sense of perspective and calm.

Instant Meditation

Here is a method for on-the-spot micro-meditation that can be used anytime, anywhere to quickly restore calm and focus. Remember to use it whenever you feel you are being overtaken by feelings of stress, anger, anxiety, or pressure.

PROCEDURE

1 Sit still, wherever you happen to be. Close your eyes.

2 Relax your body, and bring your attention to the breath.

3 Touch the tips of the first two fingers against the tip of the thumb on your right hand (or your left if you are left-handed).

4 Breathe in deeply; then breathe out slowly, while counting down from ten to zero, focusing your attention fully on each number as it comes and goes.

5 When you have reached zero, notice the difference in your state of being, and open your eyes.

6 Determine to bring this quality with you as you carry on with life.

Left: This hand position should not introduce any tension into your hand, wrist, or arm. Only the lightest of touches is necessary.

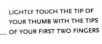

LIGHTLY TOUCH THE TIP OF YOUR THUMB WITH THE TIPS OF YOUR FIRST TWO FINGERS

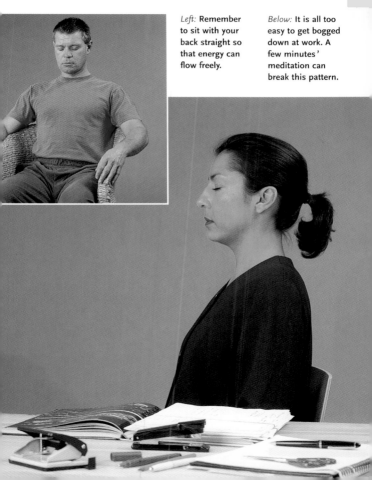

Left: **Remember to sit with your back straight so that energy can flow freely.**

Below: **It is all too easy to get bogged down at work. A few minutes' meditation can break this pattern.**

Active Meditation

Another approach to meditation is to use regular everyday
actions themselves as the focus. You can make a meditation
out of walking to work, washing the dishes, sweeping the floor,
bathing or showering, and eating. With active meditation the
notion of not having enough time to meditate is banished.

The point of active meditation is
to have awareness of the routine
activity that you are doing, rather
than being in the more common
mode – lack of attention, auto-
pilot, or daydreaming.

So the aim of the exercise is,
while eating, just to eat; while
washing the dishes, just to wash
the dishes; and so on.

• While running or walking, for
instance, you can bring your
attention to your breathing, your
heartbeat, the movement of your
limbs, and to releasing tension in
any of the muscles that are not
essential to your movement.

• Likewise when washing dishes
there is a variety of potential
focuses for the senses in all the

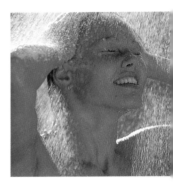

Above: You can even meditate in
the shower. Close your eyes and
focus on the sound of the water.

movements, sensations, texture:
and smells involved in eac
moment of the activity.

• When you find that your min
is wandering from the job at han(

bring it back on track. It may be helpful at such moments mentally to name the activity you are doing, such as saying to yourself "walking," "eating dinner," or "sweeping the floor."

Practicing active meditation on a regular basis during different activities will greatly improve your effectiveness in all aspects of life – as well as getting the floor or dishes cleaner than usual!

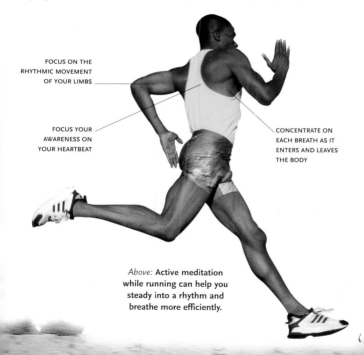

FOCUS ON THE
RHYTHMIC MOVEMENT
OF YOUR LIMBS

FOCUS YOUR
AWARENESS ON
YOUR HEARTBEAT

CONCENTRATE ON
EACH BREATH AS IT
ENTERS AND LEAVES
THE BODY

Above: **Active meditation
while running can help you
steady into a rhythm and
breathe more efficiently.**

Applying the Meditative Approach

The principles of meditation can be applied even more broadly on a moment-to-moment basis, across the whole spectrum of daily life. Doing a job with full awareness and being in the present moment, rather than with absent-mindedness or scattered focus, can be applied to almost any task in your day.

COMPONENTS OF THE MEDITATIVE APPROACH

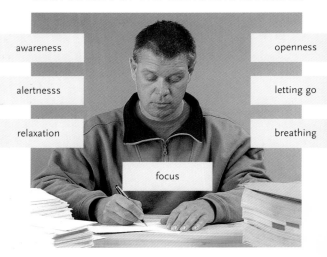

awareness

openness

alertnesss

letting go

relaxation

breathing

focus

f you apply the meditative
pproach to just a few activities
ach day, you will notice a very
efinite improvement in the
esults you are getting.

Just a moment's meditation can
elp restore calm. For example,
ou may find yourself sitting in
our car at a traffic light that
eems determined not to change to
reen, and you're not feeling at all
appy about it. While keeping
our eyes open and staying alert
o the external situation, allow
our consciousness to go into a
meditative state, or just bring your
ttention to the breath. This can
make a world of difference to the
eeling of the moment.

As you practice formal and
nformal meditation methods, you
vill find that this ability soon
pecomes second nature and begins
o pervade parts of your life
where you have not consciously
endeavored to apply it.

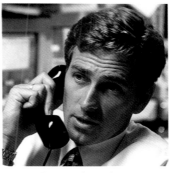

Above: Regular meditation
can help you concentrate on
the here and now.

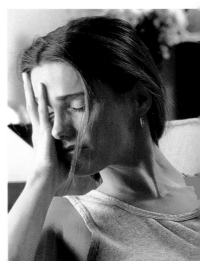

Right: Whenever you
feel stressed, close your
eyes and meditate for a
few moments.

Beyond Meditation

The benefits of meditation in improving your general health and well-being can be further enhanced by exploring a variety of other practical therapies. Here are some suggestions.

There are a number of pursuits that are traditionally associated with meditation, or can be treated as meditations in themselves. These include

- *yoga*
- *tai chi*
- *chi gung*
- *aikido*
- *dance and movement.*

There are also natural medicines and remedies that you can use yourself to help with relaxation and stress reduction, including

- herbs and herbal teas, such as camomile or peppermint
- essential oils, including lavender,

bergamot, petitgrain, neroli, and cedarwood; these can be added to a bath or used in a burner
- flower essences such as Rescue Remedy or Five Flower Remedy.

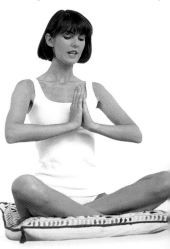

Right: **A simple position such as this can be assumed for meditative purposes.**

ESSENTIAL OILS

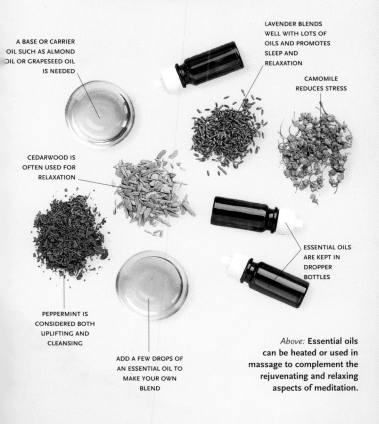

A BASE OR CARRIER
OIL SUCH AS ALMOND
OIL OR GRAPESEED OIL
IS NEEDED

LAVENDER BLENDS
WELL WITH LOTS OF
OILS AND PROMOTES
SLEEP AND
RELAXATION

CAMOMILE
REDUCES STRESS

CEDARWOOD IS
OFTEN USED FOR
RELAXATION

ESSENTIAL OILS
ARE KEPT IN
DROPPER
BOTTLES

PEPPERMINT IS
CONSIDERED BOTH
UPLIFTING AND
CLEANSING

ADD A FEW DROPS OF
AN ESSENTIAL OIL TO
MAKE YOUR OWN
BLEND

Above: Essential oils
can be heated or used in
massage to complement the
rejuvenating and relaxing
aspects of meditation.

HELPFUL DIETARY MEASURES

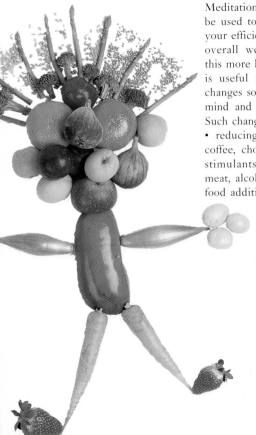

Meditation is a practice that can be used to heal yourself, increase your efficiency, and enhance your overall well-being. In line with this more healthy way of living, it is useful to make some dietary changes so that you can feed your mind and practice healthy eating. Such changes are:

• reducing your consumption of coffee, chocolate, cola, and other stimulants as well as red meat, alcohol, sugar, and artificial food additives.

• increasing your intake of fish, foods that contain vitamin A (such as carrots, apricots, broccoli, and liver), and fresh natural fruit, vegetables, and a healthy variety of wholegrains.

Left: A healthy diet filled with plenty of fruit and vegetables can enhance your powers of concentration and energize your whole being.

STRATEGIES

inally, there are certain helpful
rategies with which to approach
fe, in order to incorporate the
esults and benefits gained from
he meditative way more fully.

Whatever you are doing, try to
take one task or activity at a time.
There is nothing more debilitating
than continuously dwelling on a
whole list of things that need
doing. Instead, whether dealing
with big things or small, work out
your priorities, then start on
the top one; focus on it and set
everything else completely
aside for the time being.

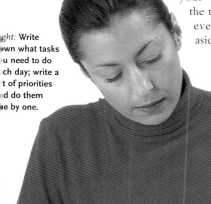

*ght: Write
wn what tasks
u need to do
ch day; write a
t of priorities
d do them
e by one.

Getting Help

It may sometimes be helpful or necessary to draw on the services of others, either to complement your meditative practice to help you get more out of it or to deal with personal issues of which you have become aware through meditation and the life changes that it can bring.

In the modern era of accessible alternative health practices, many experts in the following fields can work in ways that naturally complement meditation methods:
• bodywork, such as shiatsu and massage
• specific treatment, such as homeopathy and aromatherapy
• postural therapy, such as the Alexander Technique
• counseling.
There are also, of course, other ways of learning meditation than through books. Most cities have meditation teachers and classes, and many smaller towns do, too. See if you can find one whose methods suit you. Many of these classes also offer tapes and other aids to meditation that you can use at home to practice.

Alternatively, you could always treat yourself to a ticket to see a good comedian – laughter has a long history as a form of beneficial meditative practice!

Right: **Some people may find it much easier to learn the basic techniques as part of a class led by an experienced teacher.**

made

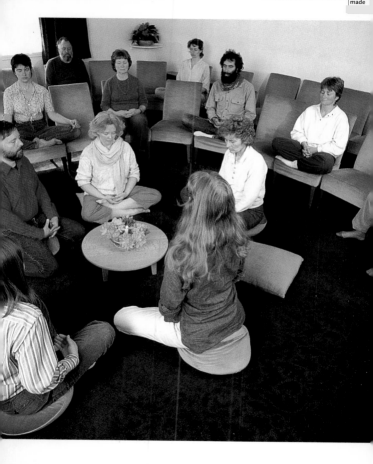

Index